I0429780

MAGNETIC
THERAPY
BENEFITS

A Complete Guide To Pain Relief,
Improved Circulation, Reduced
Inflammation, Enhanced Relaxation,
And Accelerated Healing

WILFREDO CARSON

INTRODUCTION

Magnetic therapy has arisen as a fascinating topic in alternative medicine, gaining interest for its alleged health advantages and therapeutic applications. This thorough investigation tries to shed light on the complexities of magnetic therapy, including its historical roots, theoretical foundations, and present uses. As we explore more into the issue, it becomes clear that magnetic therapy sits at the crossroads of traditional practices and modern scientific understanding, eliciting both intrigue and skepticism. This research aims to provide a thorough examination of the key concepts underlying magnetic therapy, including its historical evolution, the fundamental principles that govern its mechanisms, and the potential benefits it may offer to people looking for alternative approaches to health and well-being.

Overview of Magnetic Therapy:

Magnetic therapy, sometimes called magnotherapy, is the use of magnetic fields on the body for therapeutic purposes.

This method is based on the concept that magnets can alter the flow of energy and restore equilibrium inside the body, hence encouraging healing and easing a variety of health issues. The key concept is the interaction of magnetic fields and the body's inherent electromagnetic field, with proponents claiming that such interactions can influence biological processes at the cellular and molecular levels. As we begin our examination of magnetic therapy, it is critical to understand the many modalities used, which range from static magnets worn as jewelry to electromagnetic devices used for specific uses. According to the underlying ideas, magnetic fields can influence blood circulation, nerve conduction, and cellular metabolism, providing a non-invasive and drug-free solution to some health conditions.

Historical Background:

To understand the origins and evolution of magnetic therapy, one must go back through history. The use of magnets for healing extends back thousands of years, with ancient civilizations such as the Greeks, Egyptians, and Chinese writing their knowledge of magnetic qualities. Magnets, for example, were thought to balance the body's vital energy, or qi, in traditional Chinese medicine, whereas magnetic stones were used for their purported medicinal abilities in ancient Greece. Magnetism regained popularity throughout the Renaissance, as scientists such as Paracelsus investigated its potential applications. However, magnetic therapy gained traction in the twentieth century, with the introduction of magnetic resonance imaging (MRI) technology and the study of electromagnetic fields in medical contexts. Today, magnetic therapy combines old wisdom with current scientific investigation, motivating continuous research into its efficacy and processes.

Scope and Purpose of the Book:

This investigation into magnetic therapy goes beyond a simple examination of its historical and theoretical roots. This book covers a wide range of topics, including the scientific foundations of magnetic therapy, its current applications, and the ongoing controversies about its efficacy. Furthermore, the goal of this project is to give readers a comprehensive awareness of the potential benefits and limitations of magnetic therapy, based on empirical facts and critical analysis.

This book aims to guide readers through the complexities of magnetic therapy by examining various perspectives within the scientific community and incorporating insights from clinical studies, empowering them to make informed decisions about how to incorporate it into their health and wellness practices.

Fundamental Principles:

At the heart of magnetic therapy are fundamental principles that support its claimed benefits on the human body.

Magnetic fields, according to proponents, can alter biological processes at the cellular and molecular levels by modifying ion channels, enzyme activity, and gene expression.

One important mechanism postulated is the effect of magnetic fields on blood circulation. Magnets are thought to change the viscosity of blood, improve microcirculation, and increase oxygen supply to tissues.

Proponents also suggest that magnetic therapy may affect nerve conduction, with magnetic fields potentially affecting nerve signal transmission. These essential principles are based on the interplay of magnetic fields with the body's natural electromagnetic field, which shapes the theoretical foundation of magnetic therapy.

Potential benefits:

Exploring the potential benefits of magnetic therapy reveals a wide range of reported positive impacts on health and well-being.

One of the central claims is the role of magnetic treatment in pain management.

Magnets, according to advocates, can relieve pain by altering nerve signals, lowering inflammation, and increasing endorphin release.

This has resulted in the use of magnetic therapy for illnesses such as arthritis, migraines, and musculoskeletal discomfort. Furthermore, proponents argue that magnetic therapy may help enhance sleep quality by influencing the body's circadian cycles and melatonin synthesis.

Aside from pain relief, supporters argue that magnetic therapy can improve the healing process, increase energy levels, and contribute to overall vitality. However, these statements must be scrutinized in light of facts, as well as the current complexities and conflicts within the scientific community.

Contemporary applications:

Magnetic treatment has grown into a multifaceted field with applications in a variety of health fields. Magnetic devices such as wristbands, wraps, and insoles are marketed for their ability to relieve pain and improve overall well-being. Magnetic mattress pads and clothing accessories are intended to offer constant exposure to magnetic fields during sleep or daily activities.

Additionally, electromagnetic treatment equipment capable of producing pulsating magnetic fields is used in clinical settings to treat problems such as chronic pain and wound healing.

Magnetic treatment has been integrated into mainstream medicine, as seen by the use of transcranial magnetic stimulation (TMS) for psychiatric illnesses and the use of magnetic fields in regenerative medicine.

As we evaluate these current applications, it is critical to distinguish between anecdotal claims and scientifically validated interventions, while also acknowledging continuing research efforts to understand the processes and efficacy of magnetic therapy.

Debate and Criticism:

Magnetic therapy's entry into mainstream treatment has not been without controversy or criticism. Skeptics contend that the existing data for magnetic therapy's efficacy is contradictory and frequently characterized by methodological flaws. The placebo effect, in which people report gains due to psychological factors rather than the real treatment, is a common worry in studies on magnetic therapy. Critics underline the importance of well-designed, placebo-controlled trials in determining the genuine effects of magnetic therapy and distinguishing them from placebo responses. Furthermore, the variability of magnetic therapy devices and the lack of established protocols make it difficult to draw definitive conclusions. This section looks into the controversies and criticisms surrounding magnetic therapy, offering a balanced view of the current issues and prospective opportunities for future study in this subject.

This investigation into magnetic therapy aimed to elucidate the complexities of a practice that combines old traditions and modern scientific inquiry. Magnetic therapy presents a complex environment that requires close examination, from its historical roots to contemporary uses, fundamental principles to prospective advantages, and ongoing controversies. As people increasingly explore alternative approaches to health and well-being, understanding the nuances of magnetic therapy becomes critical. This book helps readers understand the various opinions within the scientific community, critically analyze the evidence, and make informed decisions about incorporating magnetic therapy into their healthcare practices. Magnetic treatment, whether received with curiosity or skepticism, remains a subject of continuing inquiry and exploration, adding to the larger conversation about the junction of traditional wisdom and evidence-based medicine in the goal of holistic health.

CHAPTER 1
THE FUNDAMENTALS OF MAGNETISM

Magnetism is a fundamental force in nature that is tightly woven into the fabric of our physical reality. Understanding its principles is critical for understanding the applications of magnetic therapy. Magnetism is fundamentally defined as the force of attraction or repulsion between magnetically charged things. The concept stems from the alignment of atoms within materials, which creates a magnetic field. This field is critical to realizing the potential benefits of magnetic therapy.

Understanding magnetism:

Magnetism, a discipline of physics, studies the properties and behavior of magnets. At the microscopic level, it is caused by the alignment and movement of charged particles, particularly electrons, within atoms.

The interaction of these charged particles generates a magnetic field or a zone of influence around the magnet. This field is the invisible force that causes magnetic materials to attract or repel each other. The study of magnetism entails deciphering the complexities of these atomic interactions and their macroscopic consequences for materials.

Magnetic Fields:

Magnetism is founded on the concept of magnetic field. A magnetic field is a location in space where a magnetic force can be sensed.

It emanates from a magnet's north pole and loops back to the south pole, forming a continuous closed loop. The strength of the magnetic field is measured in quantities known as Gauss or Tesla, which provide a quantitative measure of the force applied. Understanding the properties and behavior of magnetic fields is critical for realizing their therapeutic value. Magnetic therapy frequently focuses on modulating these fields to positively influence biological processes.

Types of Magnets:

Magnets are available in a variety of shapes and sizes, each with its unique qualities and applications. Permanent magnets, such as those found in compass needles, retain their magnetic qualities with time.

Temporary magnets, on the other hand, only become magnetized when subjected to a magnetic field. Electromagnets, which generate magnetic fields by sending an electric current via a wire coil, are controllable and adjustable. Understanding the subtleties of these various magnet types is critical for customizing magnetic therapy approaches to specific requirements and situations.

Magnetic polarity:

The concept of polarity is fundamental to magnetism because it defines how a magnet's north and south poles are oriented. Like poles repel and opposing poles attract.

This fundamental principle governs the alignment of magnets in therapeutic devices. Magnetic therapy relies on careful consideration of polarity to obtain the desired physiological effects. Understanding how magnetic polarity affects magnetic field behavior and interactions with the human body is critical for optimizing therapeutic approaches.

Magnetic Material:

Not all materials respond equally to magnetic fields. Ferromagnetic materials, including iron and nickel, have significant magnetic characteristics and are quickly magnetized. Paramagnetic and diamagnetic materials respond less strongly to magnetic fields. Understanding the properties of these materials is critical for developing effective magnetic treatment devices. The use of appropriate materials ensures that magnetic fields are sufficiently strong and tailored to provide therapeutic advantages.

In the field of magnetic therapy, a thorough understanding of these fundamental magnetism concepts provides the foundation for informed and effective applications.

From the complexities of magnetic fields to the various types of magnets and the importance of magnetic polarity and materials, the level of expertise directly correlates with prospective therapeutic effects.

Clinical applications of magnetic therapy:

As we explore more into the therapeutic uses of magnetic treatment, it becomes clear that the use of magnets for healing purposes has a lengthy history that spans multiple civilizations. While our scientific understanding of these applications has grown over time, magnets' therapeutic potential has been recognized in a variety of medical sectors. Examining the clinical environment indicates a wide range of possible advantages, including pain management, neurological problems, and more.

Pain Management:

Magnetic therapy has shown potential in a variety of applications, including pain control. The use of magnets to relieve pain stems from the concept that magnetic fields can impact the body's natural energy flow and restore balance. Magnetic therapy has been studied for the treatment of osteoarthritis, rheumatoid arthritis, and fibromyalgia. While the results vary, some people report less pain and a higher quality of life, encouraging more research into the mechanisms underlying these benefits.

Neurological disorders:

Magnetic therapy's impact on neurological illnesses is a developing area of research in the medical community. Transcranial magnetic stimulation (TMS) is a treatment that employs magnetic fields to activate nerve cells in the brain. TMS has shown potential in the treatment of depression, anxiety, and specific neurological illnesses. Understanding how magnetic fields interact with the nervous system is critical for improving these therapeutic techniques and applying them to a wider spectrum of neurological diseases.

Wound Healing:

Magnetic therapy has also been investigated for its possible usefulness in promoting wound healing. Magnets applied to wounds are supposed to enhance blood flow and improve nutrient and oxygen supply to the affected area.

Magnetic fields may also alter cellular functions, such as growth factor production, which can lead to faster healing. While research in this field is ongoing, preliminary data indicate that magnetic therapy may play a beneficial role in wound treatment methods.

Cardiovascular Health:

Magnetic therapy is also interested in the cardiovascular system, which has an extensive network of vessels and relies heavily on the heart. Some research has looked into the effect of magnetic fields on blood circulation, with possible benefits for illnesses like hypertension and peripheral artery disease. Understanding the physiological reactions to magnetic fields in the cardiovascular system is critical for creating targeted therapies to supplement current medical approaches.

Inflammation and Immunity Response:

The control of inflammation and immune response is a complex and crucial part of many medical diseases. Magnetic therapy has been investigated for potential anti-inflammatory effects, with some studies indicating a reduction in inflammatory markers. Understanding how magnetic fields interact with the immune system sheds light on their potential function in treating chronic inflammatory disorders.

Psychological Wellbeing:

Beyond physical health, magnetic therapy has been studied for its effects on psychological well-being. Magnetic fields' influence on neurotransmitters and brain activity has prompted research into mood disorders and stress management. Integrating knowledge of how magnetic fields affect the brain's emotional and cognitive functions is critical for establishing comprehensive approaches to mental health using magnetic treatment.

As we investigate the therapeutic applications of magnetic therapy, it becomes clear that the potential advantages span a wide range of health issues. Magnetic therapy shows potential as a supplemental technique in a variety of medical fields, ranging from pain management to neurological and cardiovascular health. Continued study and a better knowledge of the underlying mechanisms will improve the application of magnetic therapy, paving the path for novel and evidence-based treatments.

Challenges and Considerations for Magnetic Therapy:

While magnetic therapy shows promise in a variety of clinical applications, it is critical to recognize the limitations and considerations connected with its adoption. Navigating the complexities of individual responses, as well as the necessity for defined guidelines, is critical for the prudent and effective use of magnetic therapy in healthcare settings.

Individual variability:

Individual variability in reactions is one of the most critical issues in magnetic therapy. People's reactions to magnetic fields may vary depending on their age, health situation, and genetic predisposition. Understanding and accounting for this heterogeneity is critical for adapting magnetic therapy approaches to the unique needs of each individual.

Personalized techniques that take into account the various parameters determining responses can improve the efficacy of magnetic therapy while reducing the danger of side effects.

Dose-response relationships:

It is crucial to establish unambiguous dose-response connections to maximize magnetic field therapy advantages.

Magnetic field exposure can have an impact on biological systems depending on its intensity, duration, and frequency. Achieving a balance between providing an adequate therapeutic dose and preventing potential overexposure is a complex component of magnetic therapy. Research activities aimed at establishing these associations will help to develop evidence-based guidelines for the safe and successful application of magnetic therapy.

Standardization of protocols:

The absence of established protocols creates a challenge in the field of magnetic therapy. Different research may use different magnet types, configurations, and application methods, making it difficult to evaluate data and reach firm conclusions.

Establishing established protocols for magnetic therapy interventions is critical for developing a strong evidence foundation. Consistent techniques will help to replicate studies and contribute to the cumulative knowledge required to guide clinical practice.

Placebo Effects and Blindness:

The placebo effect is a crucial factor in determining magnetic treatment success.

The subjective nature of pain and other symptoms makes it difficult to determine whether benefits are due to the magnetic intervention itself or psychological reasons. Implementing strict blinding methods in clinical trials, where both participants and researchers are oblivious to the treatment status, is critical for discriminating between actual therapeutic effects and placebo reactions. This methodological rigor improves the trustworthiness of research findings and the credibility of magnetic therapy as a viable therapeutic option.

Safety Concerns:

Ensuring the safety of magnetic treatment procedures is critical. While magnetic fields are typically regarded as safe in therapeutic settings, potential hazards must be carefully examined.

High-intensity magnetic fields, particularly in devices such as transcranial magnetic stimulators, may raise safety issues.

Rigorous risk evaluations and attention to safety guidelines are required to reduce any negative effects and promote the responsible use of magnetic treatment in a variety of clinical applications.

Ethical considerations:

The ethical issues of magnetic therapy deserve careful examination. As the discipline evolves, problems may arise regarding informed consent, public knowledge dissemination, and appropriate marketing of magnetic therapy devices.

Transparency in reporting findings, accurate information to patients, and adherence to ethical norms in research and practice are critical for promoting confidence and integrity in the use of magnetic therapy.

To navigate the obstacles and considerations connected with magnetic therapy, a multidisciplinary strategy that incorporates expertise from physics, medicine, and ethics is required. By addressing individual variability, improving dose-response relationships, standardizing protocols, limiting placebo effects, assuring safety, and adhering to ethical norms, the field may move forward responsibly, maximizing the potential advantages of magnetic therapy while minimizing hazards.

Future Directions for Magnetic Therapy Research:

The landscape of magnetic therapy research is constantly changing, with current studies pushing the boundaries of knowledge and exploring new frontiers. As we look ahead, many significant topics emerge as focus points for furthering our understanding and application of magnetic therapy.

Mechanistic insights:

Future studies should focus on understanding the complexities of the mechanisms underpinning magnetic therapy's effects. Understanding magnetic fields' interactions with biological systems at the molecular, cellular, and systemic levels will yield critical insights. This understanding serves as the foundation for designing focused interventions, optimizing therapeutic techniques, and broadening the scope of illnesses for which magnetic therapy may be effective.

Bio magnetic imaging:

Advances in bio magnetic imaging technology promise to improve our ability to visualize and measure the effects of magnetic fields on the human body.

Magnetic resonance imaging (MRI) and magnetoencephalography (MEG) are two techniques that can be used to investigate the dynamic interactions of magnetic fields and tissues. Integrating bio magnetic imaging into research methods allows for real-time, non-invasive assessments, which contributes to a better understanding of the physiological reactions to magnetic therapy.

Individualized Treatment Approaches:

Precision medicine emphasizes the necessity of adapting interventions to specific patient features. Future magnetic therapy research may focus on developing tailored treatment options based on genetic, physiological, and lifestyle characteristics. Identifying biomarkers that predict individual reactions to magnetic fields might help tailor therapy procedures, improving outcomes and reducing variability in clinical research.

Combination therapies:

The synergistic effects of combining magnetic therapy with other therapeutic modalities are an interesting area for investigation. Research may look into the possible benefits of combining magnetic therapy with traditional therapies, physical therapy, or pharmacological approaches.

Understanding how magnetic therapy interacts with current medical approaches can lead to new opportunities for complete and integrated healthcare initiatives.

Long-term outcomes and safety profiles:

Long-term studies that investigate magnetic therapy's long-term effects and safety profiles are critical for determining its function in chronic disease management.

Investigating the long-term stability of therapeutic advantages and monitoring for potential adverse effects will help us gain a better understanding of magnetic therapy's risk-benefit profile.

Exploration of novel applications:

As technology progresses, new applications for magnetic therapy may arise. Nanotechnology, for example, could allow for the targeted administration of magnetic nanoparticles to specific tissues, increasing the precision of therapeutic interventions. Exploring these novel approaches necessitates interdisciplinary collaboration and a forward-thinking mindset to push the limits of what is currently achievable in the field of magnetic therapy.

Progress in magnetic treatment research will be driven by a commitment to rigorous scientific investigation, cross-disciplinary collaboration, and a focus on translating results into relevant clinical applications.

Researchers can realize magnetic therapy's full potential in promoting health and well-being by addressing mechanistic insights, leveraging bio magnetic imaging, embracing individualized treatment approaches, exploring combination therapies, assessing long-term effects, and embracing novel applications.

CHAPTER 2
MAGNETIC THERAPY EXPLAINED

Magnetic therapy, often known as magnetotherapy, is an alternative medical treatment that uses static magnets, pulsed electromagnetic fields (PEMF), or magnetic jewelry to supposedly improve health and well-being. Magnetic therapy advocates argue that the use of magnetic fields can activate numerous physiological processes within the body, resulting in therapeutic effects. Magnetic therapy has been used for centuries in numerous cultures, but its scientific basis and efficacy are still debated in the medical profession.

Definition and Principles of Magnetic Therapy:

Magnetic treatment is based on the idea that exposure to magnetic fields might alter the body's electromagnetic balance, potentially leading to therapeutic effects.

Proponents argue that the human body produces its electromagnetic field and that changes to this field can contribute to a variety of health disorders. Magnetic therapy seeks to restore or rebalance these electromagnetic forces by using magnets or magnetic fields externally. The basic notion is that magnetic energy enters the body and interacts with cells, tissues, and nerves to promote healing and relieve symptoms.

The fundamental ideas of magnetic therapy frequently rely on the concept of biomagnetism, which holds that the body's cells and tissues contain magnetic materials and respond to external magnetic fields. This contact is hypothesized to influence cellular activities, including ion exchange, circulation, and neurotransmitter release. However, it is important to highlight that, while there is some scientific evidence indicating the presence of magnetic minerals in the body, the precise mechanisms by which magnetic therapy exerts its benefits are unknown and require further investigation.

How Magnetic Therapy Works:

Magnetic therapy is thought to work in a variety of ways, while the specifics are unknown. One hypothesized explanation is based on magnetic fields' effects on ion channels and cell membranes. Proponents say that magnetic fields influence the passage of ions across cell membranes, modifying electrical charge and, as a result, cellular processes. This, in turn, is thought to affect processes such as nerve transmission, muscle contraction, and hormone release.

Another proposed mechanism is the circulation of blood. Magnetic therapy supporters believe that magnets can improve blood flow by dilating blood vessels and increasing oxygen and nutrient delivery to tissues. Improved circulation is supposed to help with the healing process and minimize inflammation. However, scientific studies looking into these claims have generated varied findings, with some indicating potential advantages and others finding no meaningful impacts.

Furthermore, magnetic therapy is frequently linked to altered pain perception. It is hypothesized that magnetic fields can impact the transmission of pain signals in the neurological system, resulting in pain alleviation. This concept is based on the gate control hypothesis of pain, which states that non-painful stimuli, such as magnets, can block the "gate" to painful stimuli, reducing pain perception. However, the therapeutic efficacy of magnetic treatment for pain management is still being studied and debated.

Types of Magnetic Therapy:

Magnetic therapy involves a variety of treatments, each using distinct types of magnetic fields for therapeutic objectives. These include static magnets, PEMF therapy, and magnetic jewelry.

Static Magnets:

Static magnets are arguably the most frequent type of magnetic therapy. These are stationary magnets that can be worn directly on the skin or concealed within clothing and accessories. Proponents say that constant exposure to static magnetic fields can provide a variety of health benefits, including pain alleviation and enhanced sleep.

Despite their popularity, the scientific evidence for static magnets' usefulness is inconsistent. While some studies show good results, others discover no meaningful difference between using static magnets and a placebo.

Pulsed Electromagnetic Field (PEMF) Treatment:

PEMF therapy uses electromagnetic fields that vary in intensity and frequency over time.

Unlike static magnets, PEMF devices generate pulsating magnetic fields that are considered to reach deeper into tissues. Advocates of PEMF therapy claim that it can increase cellular activity, improve healing, and reduce inflammation.

Some research backs up the efficacy of PEMF therapy in specific applications including bone repair and pain control. However, further research is required to determine its efficacy in a broader spectrum of illnesses.

Magnetic Jewelry:

Magnetic jewelry, such as bracelets, necklaces, and rings, incorporate magnets into their design, allowing for constant, low-level exposure to magnetic fields. Wearing magnetic jewelry, according to proponents, can give continuing therapeutic benefits, such as addressing pain, stiffness, and weariness. Magnetic jewellery's convenience and non-invasive nature make it popular among people looking for alternative health remedies.

While some users report subjective advantages, scientific data supporting the usefulness of magnetic jewelry is sparse and warrants further investigation.

Magnetic therapy is still a source of curiosity and controversy in the field of alternative medicine. Despite centuries of use and anecdotal evidence of benefits, the scientific community still does not completely understand the mechanisms by which magnetic therapy works.

The current study yields varied results, with some studies indicating potential benefits in specific situations and others finding no substantial influence beyond a placebo effect. As research in this subject progress, a more complete understanding of magnetic therapy's principles, methods, and efficacy may emerge, offering information on its potential role in integrative medicine.

CHAPTER 3
BENEFITS OF MAGNETIC THERAPY

Pain Management:

Magnetic treatment has attracted attention for its potential benefits in pain management, as it provides a non-invasive alternative to alleviating various forms of pain.

Magnetic therapy has shown tremendous promise in the treatment of arthritis. Arthritis, which is characterized by joint inflammation, stiffness, and discomfort, can provide substantial issues for people. Magnetic therapy is thought to work by altering the movement of ions and electrons in affected areas, modifying pain signals, and lowering inflammation. Research studies have looked into the use of magnetic devices, such as bracelets or pads, to provide relief to arthritis patients, demonstrating magnetic therapy's potential as a supplemental pain treatment.

Furthermore, magnetic therapy has shown success in treating musculoskeletal pain, which includes disorders such as back pain, neck pain, and joint discomfort.

Magnetic fields are hypothesized to improve blood flow, promote endorphin release, and potentially modify nerve signaling, all of which help with pain alleviation. Chronic pain disorders, which frequently provide long-term challenges for patients, have also been a focus of magnetic treatment research. According to studies, magnetic therapy may play a role in changing pain perceptions and fostering a more sustainable approach to pain management than typical pharmacological approaches.

Improved blood circulation:

Magnetic therapy has a significant physiological effect that improves blood circulation. Proper blood flow is essential for delivering oxygen and nutrients to different tissues and organs throughout the body. Magnetic fields are thought to alter ion exchange within blood arteries, causing vasodilation and increased blood flow.

This effect is especially essential in situations when poor blood circulation causes symptoms or problems. According to research, magnetic therapy may benefit people with vascular problems including peripheral artery disease by increasing vasodilation and improving blood circulation to affected areas. Furthermore, improved blood circulation may allow for more efficient elimination of metabolic waste products, benefiting overall tissue health and function.

Inflammation reduction:

Magnetic therapy's anti-inflammatory capabilities have piqued the curiosity of clinicians and researchers alike. Inflammation is a prevalent factor in a variety of health disorders, including acute traumas and chronic diseases. Magnetic fields are hypothesized to regulate inflammatory processes by affecting cellular signaling pathways. Studies have investigated the effect of magnetic therapy on inflammatory markers, revealing potential reductions in pro-inflammatory chemicals. This anti-inflammatory action may have ramifications for disorders like rheumatoid arthritis, where chronic inflammation causes joint destruction. Understanding the methods by which magnetic therapy interacts with inflammatory pathways sheds light on its therapeutic potential and function in reducing the negative effects of chronic inflammation.

Improved Sleep Quality:

Magnetic therapy has been linked to improved sleep quality, offering a non-pharmacological option for people suffering from sleep disorders or disruptions.

Sleep is vital for overall health and well-being since it affects cognitive performance, emotional management, and immune system function. Magnetic fields are thought to influence the generation of melatonin, which regulates the sleep-wake cycle. Magnetic therapy, which modulates melatonin levels, may help to build a more consistent and peaceful sleep pattern. Magnetic mattress pads or sleep masks have been studied for their ability to improve sleep quality, particularly in people suffering from insomnia or circadian rhythm abnormalities.

Understanding the influence of magnetic therapy on sleep systems opens a new option for managing sleep-related disorders without the risks associated with pharmacological interventions.

Stress & Anxiety Relief:

Magnetic therapy has been studied in the field of mental health for its ability to relieve tension and anxiety. Stress and anxiety disorders are common in modern life, affecting both mental and physical health.

Magnetic fields are hypothesized to impact neurotransmitter activity and hormone balance, leading to a more relaxed physiological state.

According to research, magnetic therapy may reduce stress hormone levels, such as cortisol, while increasing the release of neurotransmitters like serotonin and endorphins.

These neurotransmitters are important for mood regulation and overall well-being. Magnetic therapy devices, ranging from magnetic jewelry to customized mats, have been studied as methods for treating stress and anxiety.

Understanding the neurological mechanisms that underpin these effects provides important insights into the possible integration of magnetic treatment into mental health interventions.

Accelerated healing:

The concept of rapid healing with magnetic therapy is based on the premise that magnetic fields can positively influence cellular processes involved in tissue repair and regeneration. The biological response to magnetic fields is extensive and varied, involving interactions with numerous signaling pathways. Magnetic treatment has been studied for its effect on the proliferation and differentiation of wound-healing cells such as fibroblasts and endothelial cells. Magnetic fields may also influence the release of growth factors and cytokines, which play critical roles in tissue regeneration.

The possibility for rapid healing applies to a wide range of ailments, including musculoskeletal injuries, fractures, and post-surgical recovery.

As researchers continue to untangle intricate biological mechanics, magnetic treatment shows potential as a complementary strategy to enhancing the body's natural healing processes.

Magnetic therapy has numerous health benefits, including pain control and increased blood circulation, as well as inflammation reduction, improved sleep quality, stress and anxiety relief, and faster recovery. Understanding the underlying physiological principles and the various uses of magnetic therapy lays the groundwork for its incorporation into holistic healthcare models.

While more research is needed to determine particular dosages, treatment durations, and appropriate application methods, the available evidence suggests that magnetic therapy can make substantial contributions to both preventative and therapeutic healthcare initiatives. As the field evolves, the potential for magnetic treatment to supplement established interventions and increase general well-being is still being investigated and researched.

CHAPTER 4
SCIENTIFIC EVIDENCE AND RESEARCH

Magnetic therapy, often known as magnet therapy or magnotherapy, has been the focus of scientific research to better understand its potential health effects. The study of magnetic therapy entails a thorough investigation of the effects of magnetic fields on biological systems. Numerous researches has looked into the potential mechanisms underlying magnetic therapy, specifically how magnetic fields can alter various physiological processes. Researchers have looked into how magnetic fields affect cellular activity, neuron conduction, blood flow, and general body balance. Scientists have conducted in vitro and in vivo research to identify the molecular and cellular processes through which magnetic therapy may exert its effects.

An Overview of Magnetic Therapy Studies

A comprehensive review of magnetic therapy research indicates a wide spectrum of studies from several fields, including physics, medicine, and biology. Early studies concentrated on understanding the fundamental principles of magnetism and how it interacts with biological tissues.

As technology advanced, researchers looked into the development of magnetic devices for therapy, such as magnets and magnetic bracelets. Magnetic therapy has been investigated for its use in the treatment of a variety of health issues, including pain and inflammation, as well as neurological abnormalities.

The breadth of these investigations illustrates the interdisciplinary character of magnetic therapy research, which draws on expertise in physics, engineering, and medical sciences.

Clinical trials and findings

Clinical studies are an essential component of determining the efficacy and safety of magnetic therapy in real-world settings.

These trials use human subjects and rigorous procedures to evaluate the effects of magnetic therapies on certain health outcomes.

Clinical trials have been done to assess the efficacy of magnetic therapy in illnesses such as chronic pain, arthritis, and wound healing. The findings of these trials shed light on magnetic therapy's possible therapeutic benefits. However, interpreting results is not always easy, and variables such as study design, participant characteristics, and placebo effects have been scrutinized.

Criticism and Controversy

Despite the rising corpus of data on magnetic therapy, it has not been without criticism and debate. Skeptics say that the scientific evidence supporting the efficacy of magnetic therapy is uneven and frequently lacking in methodological rigor. Critics argue that many studies have limited sample sizes, poor blinding, and a lack of established methodologies. The placebo effect is also a major worry, as people may perceive benefits from magnetic therapy based on psychological variables rather than the magnetic fields themselves. Furthermore, disagreements exist over the ideal strength and duration of magnetic exposure required for therapeutic effects, complicating the interpretation of study results.

Future Research Directions

As the field of magnetic therapy evolves, future studies will strive to fill knowledge gaps and improve our grasp of its mechanics and uses. Advances in imaging techniques, such as functional magnetic resonance imaging (fMRI) and magnetic resonance spectroscopy, allow researchers to investigate the effects of magnetic fields on brain function and biochemistry. Researchers are also looking at combining magnetic therapy with other treatment methods, such as standard pharmacotherapy or physical therapy, to improve overall clinical outcomes. Wearable magnetic devices and targeted magnetic field delivery systems are another area of investigation.

Future research should focus on large-scale, well-designed clinical trials to give strong evidence and overcome doubts about magnetic therapy's efficacy.

Scientific data and research in the field of magnetic therapy have advanced significantly, with studies ranging from basic principles to clinical trials. While some studies indicate possible advantages, objections, and debates remain, needing cautious study design and interpretation. Future research areas show promise for resolving the complexities of magnetic therapy and establishing its place in mainstream healthcare.

CHAPTER 5
APPLICATIONS OF MAGNETIC THERAPY

Magnetic therapy has generated interest and investigation due to its possible health advantages. This type of alternative medicine is based on the idea that exposure to magnetic fields might have a therapeutic effect on the body. While the scientific community continues to investigate the principles underlying magnetic therapy, proponents believe it can impact the body's inherent electromagnetic fields to promote healing and alleviate a variety of health issues. In this comprehensive discussion, we will look at the numerous applications of magnetic therapy, including magnetic wristbands, beds, insoles, and wraps. We will also examine criteria for safe and successful use, as well as how magnetic therapy might be integrated into traditional medicine.

The use of magnetic therapy devices is an important component of this alternative therapeutic technique. Magnetic bracelets, for example, are worn gadgets that are said to give constant exposure to magnetic fields. Advocates say that these magnetic fields may improve blood circulation, reduce inflammation, and boost overall health.

While some studies reveal possible benefits, the scientific community is still divided on the effectiveness of magnetic bracelets, highlighting the need for more research to generate definitive evidence.

Magnetic mattresses are another type of magnetic therapy device.

These magnetized mattresses are intended to be used regularly. Proponents believe that the magnetic fields emitted by these mattresses can improve sleep quality, alleviate discomfort, and speed up the body's healing processes. However, robust scientific research is required to test these claims and identify the particular processes by which magnetic mattresses may exert their potential effects.

Magnetic insoles, which are frequently incorporated into footwear, are thought to activate acupressure points on the feet, impacting a variety of physiological activities. Advocates claim that these insoles can alleviate diseases such as foot discomfort, arthritis, and even back problems. Despite anecdotal reports of increased comfort, scientific proof for the effectiveness of magnetic insoles is lacking. Research in this area is critical for understanding the physiological impact of magnetic fields on the feet and their potential to influence general health.

Magnetic wraps, placed around specific body regions, are intended to target specific areas of pain or damage. Magnetic wraps, which are commonly used to treat diseases such as joint pain and muscle injuries, seek to harness the alleged therapeutic capabilities of magnetic fields. Studies on the efficacy of magnetic wraps have yielded varied results, with some indicating possible benefits in pain treatment. However, given the heterogeneity in study designs and the necessity for bigger, well-controlled trials, these findings should be interpreted with caution.

Guidelines for safe and successful use are critical in ensuring that people seeking magnetic therapy reap the advantages without suffering side effects. It is critical to evaluate the intensity and duration of magnetic exposure, as well as the individual's health status. While magnetic therapy is usually regarded as safe for most people, those with particular medical conditions, such as pacemakers or pregnancy, should exercise caution and seek medical advice before utilizing magnetic therapy devices.

Magnetic therapy's integration with conventional medicine is a complex and continuous process. While some proponents argue for magnetic therapy's integration into mainstream treatment, a lack of strong scientific proof presents hurdles. Collaboration between practitioners of conventional medicine and proponents of magnetic therapy is required to bridge the gap between these two approaches.

Research into the compatibility, safety, and potential synergies between magnetic therapy and conventional therapies is required for informed and evidence-based healthcare decisions.

Magnetic treatment, which includes gadgets such as wristbands, beds, insoles, and wraps, is an exciting but contentious topic in alternative medicine. The potential benefits of magnetic therapy are frequently anecdotal, and scientific evidence supporting its usefulness is still inconclusive. As research in this area develops, it is crucial to approach magnetic treatment with a critical perspective, acknowledging the importance of well-designed trials in determining its genuine therapeutic potential. Guidelines for safe use and collaboration with traditional medicine are critical issues to consider in the current research into magnetic treatment as a complementary or alternative approach to health and wellness.

CHAPTER 6
CONDITIONS AND AILMENTS

Magnetic therapy has gained popularity as a viable alternative or supplement to traditional medical treatments for a variety of illnesses and ailments. Magnetic therapy's core theory is based on the interaction between the body and magnetic fields, with proponents claiming that exposure to certain magnetic fields can improve biological processes. While the scientific community is divided on the efficacy of magnetic therapy, there is a growing amount of research looking into its potential advantages for specific ailments.

This conversation dives into the use of magnetic therapy for migraines and headaches, back pain, sleeplessness, fibromyalgia, and sports injuries.

Specific ailments and magnetic therapy

Migraines & Headaches

Migraines and headaches are common neurological illnesses that can have a major influence on patients' quality of life. Magnetic treatment has been offered as a non-pharmacological technique to help reduce the frequency and intensity of these episodes. Magnetic therapy advocates believe that applying magnetic fields to the head can modify neuronal activity and reduce the frequency of migraines or headaches.

Some research has looked into the effectiveness of transcranial magnetic stimulation (TMS), a type of magnetic therapy, in migraine management.

TMS is the application of powerful magnetic fields to activate or inhibit nerve cells in the brain. While research is ongoing, preliminary data suggest that TMS may help alleviate migraine symptoms by modulating cortical excitability.

Back Pain.

Millions of people worldwide suffer from chronic back pain, which is both common and debilitating. Magnetic therapy has been investigated as a potential non-invasive, drug-free treatment for back pain.

Magnets are thought to improve blood circulation and reduce inflammation, so alleviating pain. Proponents also suggest that magnetic therapy may influence the creation of endorphins, the body's natural painkillers, offering additional relief to people suffering from chronic back pain. However, it is important to highlight that the scientific evidence supporting the efficacy of magnetic therapy for back pain is ambiguous, with some studies indicating benefits and others reporting no significant difference when compared to a placebo.

Insomnia

Insomnia, defined as difficulty falling or staying asleep, can have serious consequences for both mental and physical health. Magnetic therapy, including the use of magnetic mattress pads or sleep masks, has been recommended as a non-pharmacological strategy for improving sleep. Advocates argue that magnetic fields may alter the generation of melatonin, a hormone important for regulating sleep-wake cycles. Additionally, magnetic therapy's soothing effects on the nervous system are thought to contribute to better sleep quality. While some people report beneficial results with magnetic therapy for insomnia, the scientific data is weak, and more thorough research is needed to demonstrate its efficacy as a reliable sleep aid.

Fibromyalgia

Fibromyalgia is a complicated chronic pain disorder characterized by widespread musculoskeletal discomfort, tiredness, and sleep disruption. Some people with fibromyalgia use alternative therapies, such as magnetic therapy, to control their symptoms. Magnetic wristbands, wraps, and mats are frequently utilized in the idea that they help relieve pain and enhance overall health. Magnetic therapy, according to proponents, may improve the body's energy flow and balance, lowering pain and discomfort caused by fibromyalgia. However, limited scientific data supports the use of magnetic therapy for fibromyalgia, and a more rigorous study is required to evaluate its efficacy and mechanisms of action.

Sports Injuries.

Athletes frequently sustain numerous injuries and seek novel techniques for rehabilitation and pain treatment. Magnetic therapy has developed as a promising supplementary treatment for sports injuries, to accelerate healing and relieve pain. Magnets, according to proponents, can improve blood flow, reduce inflammation, and stimulate tissue repair. Furthermore, magnetic therapy is thought to have analgesic properties, providing pain relief without the adverse effects associated with conventional pain drugs. While some studies suggest that magnetic therapy may be beneficial for specific sports injuries, the overall body of evidence is insufficient to draw clear conclusions. More study is needed to determine the appropriate parameters for magnetic therapy in sports injury rehabilitation and its incorporation into overall treatment strategies.

Magnetic therapy is an intriguing field with potential applications for a variety of disorders and illnesses. The scientific community is still investigating the causes and efficacy of magnetic therapy, and while some encouraging findings have been reported, a more thorough study is required to establish its presence in mainstream medical practice. Individuals seeking magnetic therapy should approach it with caution and knowledge, understanding that its efficacy may vary depending on the ailment and individual. As with any alternative therapy, interaction with healthcare professionals is required to ensure that magnetic therapy supplements rather than replaces evidence-based medical therapies.

CHAPTER 7
PERSONAL STORIES AND TESTIMONIALS.

Magnetic therapy has grown in popularity in recent years, and personal experiences and testimonials have a significant impact on public perception and comprehension of its potential advantages. Real-life experiences with magnetic therapy frequently illustrate the subjective nature of its effects, with people expressing their paths and conclusions.

These stories offer significant insights into the various ways people use magnetic therapy in their lives, whether for pain relief, better sleep, or overall well-being.

Success Stories:

Success stories about magnetic therapy abound, indicating a wide range of beneficial outcomes reported by people who have included this alternative strategy in their healthcare practice.

Many people attribute relief from chronic pain, such as arthritis or migraines, to the use of magnetic therapy. Success stories frequently emphasize magnetic therapy's holistic aspect, implying that it can enhance not only physical health but also mental and emotional well-being.

These stories add to the growing body of anecdotal data demonstrating the effectiveness of magnetic therapy as a supplemental or alternative health intervention.

Challenges and limitations:

While magnetic therapy has received much appreciation for its potential advantages, it is critical to investigate the problems and limitations connected with its implementation. Some people may report little or no improvement in their illness, raising concerns about the efficacy of magnetic therapy in general.

Furthermore, the lack of standardized guidelines for magnetic treatment applications creates issues in terms of consistency and reliability. Understanding magnetic therapy's limits is critical for setting realistic expectations and guiding future research efforts to improve and optimize its use.

Personal anecdotes and testimonials are an important part of the discussion surrounding magnetic therapy, putting light on the many experiences people have had with this alternative approach. Success stories add to the expanding body of evidence supporting magnetic therapy's potential advantages, while an examination of problems and limitations yields a more nuanced understanding of its scope and applicability.

CHAPTER 8
PRECAUTIONS AND CONTRAINDICATIONS

Magnetic treatment has grown in popularity as a non-invasive, alternative technique to improving health and well-being.

However, like with any form of therapy, it is critical to be aware of the risks and contraindications connected with magnetic therapy. Individuals with particular medical disorders or who use specific medical devices should take caution when attempting magnetic therapy. Pregnant women, people with pacemakers, and those with implanted medical equipment, such as insulin pumps, should avoid magnetic therapy or use it with caution. Furthermore, people with illnesses such as epilepsy or hemophilia should check with their doctors before undergoing magnetic therapy. These considerations underline the need to adapt magnetic therapy to individual health situations, as well as the need for a complete assessment before initiation.

Who Should Avoid Magnetic Therapy?

While magnetic therapy is generally regarded as safe for most people, some should proceed with caution or avoid it entirely.

Pregnant women, particularly those in the first trimester, should exercise caution due to a lack of extensive studies on the potential effects of magnetic fields on fetal development. Individuals with pacemakers or other implanted electronic devices may be susceptible to interference from intense magnetic fields, which could impair the proper functioning of these devices.

Furthermore, persons with metal implants, such as joint replacements, may feel discomfort or heat in the presence of intense magnetic fields.

Those with sensitive skin or allergies to specific materials used in magnetic items should exercise caution to avoid skin discomfort. Understanding these factors is critical to assuring the safety and efficacy of magnetic therapy in various populations.

Potential Risks and Side Effects:

While magnetic therapy is generally considered safe, it is critical to recognize the risks and adverse effects associated with its use. One of the most pressing issues is the likelihood of interference with electronic medical devices such as pacemakers or insulin pumps.

The magnetic fields produced by therapeutic magnets may disturb the operation of these devices, providing a risk to people who have such implants. Furthermore, continuous exposure to intense magnetic fields can cause localized heating in tissues, potentially resulting in discomfort or burns.

It is critical to utilize magnetic therapy products as advised and prevent excessive or prolonged exposure. Some people may also experience minor adverse effects, such as skin irritation or allergic responses, especially if they are sensitive to the materials used in magnetic devices. While the hazards are generally modest, knowing and limiting them are critical components of responsible magnetic treatment use.

Consultation with Health Professionals:

Before starting a magnetic therapy regimen, consumers should consult with a healthcare expert. Healthcare providers know to evaluate a patient's overall health, medical history, and potential contraindications that may affect the suitability of magnetic therapy.

A thorough assessment enables healthcare providers to detect any underlying diseases or medical equipment that could interfere with magnetic therapy. Individuals with cardiovascular concerns or a history of seizures, for example, may require specific magnetic therapy recommendations. Additionally, pregnant women seeking magnetic therapy should consult with their obstetricians to assure the safety of both the mother and the developing fetus.

The involvement of healthcare professionals in the decision-making process ensures that magnetic therapy is customized to individual health needs and reduces the dangers connected with its use.

While magnetic treatment provides a non-invasive and alternative approach to wellness, it is critical to understand the precautions, contraindications, potential hazards, and the importance of talking with healthcare specialists before adopting it into one's health regimen. Understanding the many groups of people who should exercise caution or avoid magnetic therapy entirely, such as pregnant women, those with implanted devices, and those with certain medical conditions, is critical for promoting responsible and safe use. Recognizing potential hazards and side effects, such as interference with electrical equipment or localized heating, highlights the need to follow directions and receive proper supervision when using magnetic therapy products. Finally, collaborating with healthcare specialists ensures that magnetic therapy is tailored to individual health situations while reducing potential dangers.

CHAPTER 9
CHOOSING THE RIGHT MAGNETIC THERAPY PRODUCT

Choosing the right magnetic treatment product is an important part of maximizing the potential benefits of this alternative healing method. When making this decision, several variables are considered to ensure that the chosen product meets the needs and preferences of the individual. First, the strength of the magnetic field emitted by the therapeutic device must be considered.

The strength is frequently measured in Gauss, and it is critical to select a product with the appropriate magnetic strength for the intended therapeutic purpose. For example, greater Gauss values may be appropriate for deep tissue penetration, whilst lower values may be preferred for more superficial uses.

Furthermore, the shape and form of the magnetic therapy device have a considerable impact on its effectiveness. Magnetic jewelry, wraps, cushions, and beds are among the many goods available on the market. The decision is based on the area of the body to be treated and personal comfort preferences. Magnetic wraps or pads may be better suited for localized conditions like joint discomfort, but magnetic mattresses provide a comprehensive approach to total wellness. It is critical to examine the product's simplicity and practicality to ensure constant use, as adhering to the suggested therapy regimen is essential for attaining optimal outcomes.

Factors To Consider:

When it comes to magnetic therapy, there are numerous aspects to consider that might have a big impact on the treatment's efficacy. To begin, the individual's health status and the specific ailment they wish to address should be thoroughly reviewed. Magnetic treatment devices address a variety of health conditions, including pain reduction, increased circulation, and overall well-being. Understanding the individual's demands and goals is critical in determining the best magnetic therapy technique.

Furthermore, the length and frequency of use are critical to getting the intended results. Some magnetic therapy items are intended for constant usage, while others may be indicated for occasional use. Decisions about the duration and frequency of application should be guided by factors such as the magnetic field's strength and the therapy's intended goal. Consulting with healthcare specialists or magnetic therapy experts might provide useful information for personalizing the treatment approach to individual needs.

Quality and Safety Standards:

Ensuring the quality and safety of magnetic treatment products is critical to their effectiveness and the well-being of those who use them. Quality standards include a variety of factors, such as the materials used in the product's construction, the longevity of the magnets, and overall craftsmanship.

It is critical to choose products that meet recognized quality requirements, as they assure the longevity and dependability of the magnetic therapy device.

Safety precautions are critical, as magnetic fields can interact with certain medical conditions or gadgets. Individuals with pacemakers, for example, should exercise caution while utilizing magnetic treatment items because the magnetic fields may interfere with the operation of such medical devices. As a result, selecting products with clear safety rules and recommendations is critical. Furthermore, adherence to legal standards and certifications, such as ISO (International Organization for Standardization) certifications, ensures product quality and safety.

Review and Recommendations:

In today's internet age, user evaluations and recommendations are critical in directing people to reliable and successful magnetic therapy goods.

Access to online forums where users share their experiences with specific items can provide useful information about the real-world effectiveness of magnetic therapy equipment. Analyzing a wide range of reviews enables prospective customers to assess the product's performance across different individuals and health circumstances.

However, reviews must be approached with a critical perspective, taking into account aspects such as the source's legitimacy and the regularity of criticism. Reviews from qualified health professionals or magnetic treatment experts are more credible than anecdotal accounts that lack a scientific basis.

Furthermore, requesting recommendations from healthcare specialists or practitioners who specialize in magnetic therapy can provide individualized advice based on specific health profiles.

The decision to purchase a magnetic therapy product requires careful consideration and research. Considerations like as product strength and design, individual health conditions, quality and safety requirements, and user feedback all contribute to a complete strategy for optimizing magnetic therapy's potential advantages. As the field evolves, staying up to date on breakthroughs and collaborating with healthcare specialists provides a personalized and effective magnetic therapy experience for anyone seeking alternative treatment approaches.

CHAPTER 10
INTEGRATING MAGNETIC THERAPY INTO YOUR LIFESTYLE

<u>Incorporating Magnetic Therapy into Daily Life:</u>

Magnetic treatment, a centuries-old procedure, is gaining popularity today. The concept relies on the use of magnetic fields on the body to promote healing and overall well-being. Integrating magnetic therapy into one's everyday practice necessitates a thorough understanding of the principles and potential advantages. The basic idea is that magnets can affect the body's electromagnetic field, consequently altering numerous physiological processes. Individuals can efficiently utilize magnetic therapy by using magnetic bracelets, mattress mats, or magnetic wraps. These can be worn or employed in regular activities, providing constant exposure to magnetic fields. However, moderation is essential, since excessive or incorrect use may give unsatisfactory results and may pose hazards. When adding magnetic treatment into your everyday routine, keep your specific needs, preferences, and any underlying health concerns in mind.

Complementary therapies:

Magnetic therapy is frequently seen as a complementary method to traditional medical therapies. It is critical to understand its role in conjunction with other therapies to maximize possible benefits. Magnetic therapy can supplement traditional therapies by targeting many elements of health and well-being.

For instance, it may be used alongside physical therapy to reduce discomfort and enhance the healing process. Additionally, integrating magnetic treatment with stress reduction approaches, such as meditation or acupuncture, may contribute to a more holistic approach to health. However, it is necessary to speak with healthcare professionals before integrating magnetic therapy with other treatments, ensuring that there are no contraindications or potential harmful effects. The synergy between magnetic therapy and complementary approaches highlights the importance of a multidimensional approach to health care.

Long-Term Considerations:

When contemplating the integration of magnetic therapy into one's lifestyle, considering the long-term implications is crucial. While short-term benefits may be evident, understanding the sustained impact on health is essential. Long-term considerations involve assessing the durability of magnetic products, their maintenance, and potential adjustments to the therapy over time. It is also imperative to stay informed about emerging research and advancements in magnetic therapy to adapt practices accordingly. Moreover, individuals should be aware of any changes in their health status and adjust the magnetic therapy regimen accordingly. Regular check-ups with healthcare professionals can provide valuable insights into the effectiveness of magnetic therapy over the long term and help make informed decisions about its continuation. Balancing short-term relief with long-term health goals is integral to maximizing the benefits of magnetic therapy.

CONCLUSION

the incorporation of magnetic therapy into daily routines offers a fascinating avenue for enhancing overall well-being.

By understanding the principles of magnetic therapy and its potential benefits, individuals can make informed decisions about its integration into their lifestyles.

The concept of incorporating magnetic therapy into daily routines involves judicious use of magnetic products, considering individual needs, and avoiding excessive or inappropriate applications. Furthermore, recognizing magnetic therapy as a complementary approach to conventional treatments underscores its potential to enhance various aspects of health and healing. However, this integration should be approached with caution, consulting healthcare professionals to ensure compatibility with existing treatments and avoid potential contraindications.

The long-term considerations associated with magnetic therapy highlight the need for a sustainable approach. Individuals should be mindful of the durability and maintenance of magnetic products, stay informed about evolving research, and adapt their practices over time. Regular communication with healthcare professionals becomes paramount in assessing the sustained impact of magnetic therapy on health. The synergy between short-term relief and long-term health goals becomes evident, emphasizing the importance of a balanced and informed approach to maximize the benefits of magnetic therapy.

In essence, magnetic therapy presents an intriguing dimension to holistic well-being. While it may not replace conventional medical treatments, its potential as a complementary therapy should not be overlooked.

The integration of magnetic therapy into daily routines requires a nuanced understanding, and its benefits are best realized when approached with moderation, awareness, and a commitment to long-term health.